SUPPORTING
PTSD
RECOVERY

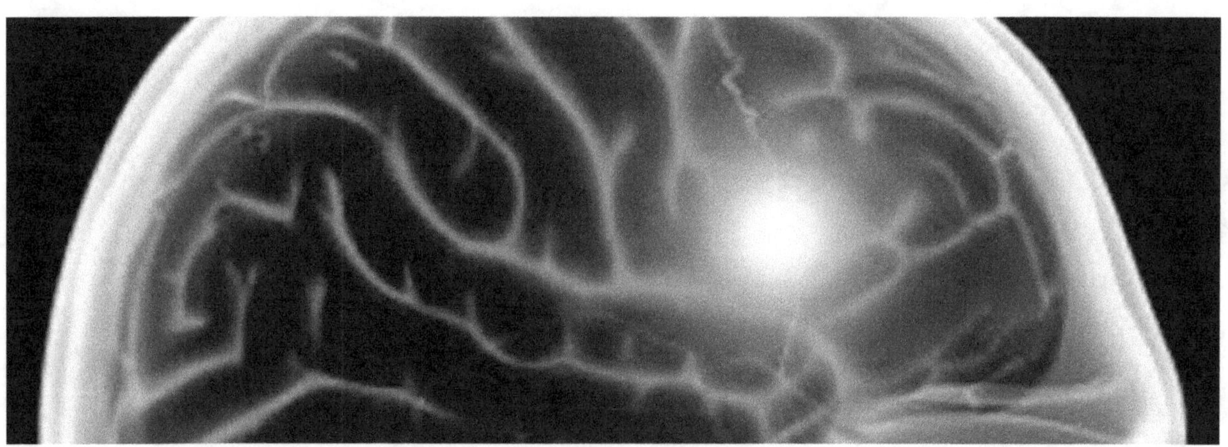

Post Traumatic Stress Disorder (PTSD) and every other neurological challenge is caused by or accentuated by misfolding of the proteins. We have learned through Glycoscience how to better fold the proteins.

JC SPENCER

To integrate proven methods to conquer PTSD with any traditional practice may be acceptable; but to integrate multiple proven methods with Glycoscience proves to be more effective.

ISBN-13 978-1717287588
ISBN-10 1717287581

In honor of all whom have been impacted by trauma. May friends and family understand and gather around to assist in overcoming the negative with solutions.

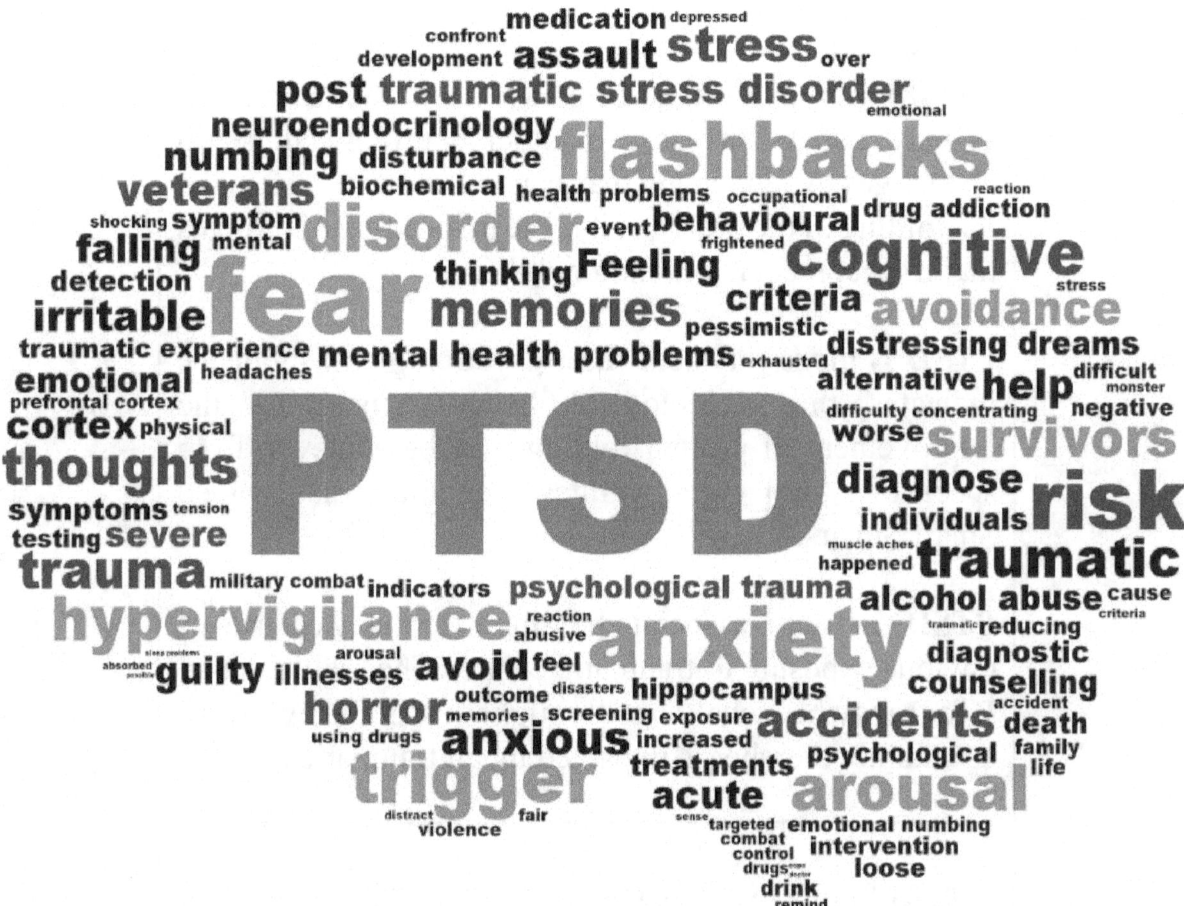

None of us like to admit that we have a "disorder." A very small "out of order" IS a "Disorder." If even a little PTSD is evident in any of us and the "D" does not stand for "Disorder" – it may stand for "Denial." Wanting to feel better is a PTSD trait. My friend Curtis Brown calls PTSD, *"Programmed To Self Destruct."*

PTSD is normally triggered by a sudden traumatic event as may also be the case in other neurological health challenges. A sudden jolt may cause a massive shift in the misfolding of the proteins. It is the misfolding of proteins that impact mental and motor skills.

PTSD is more physical than psychological. Evidence indicates that neurological benefits including the improvement of protein folding may be achieved from specific natural carbohydrates the author has named Smart Sugars.

PTSD is often associated with Veterans because of obvious exposure to traumatic events. The reality is that **PTSD** may be a challenge throughout all of us when we or a family member is impacted by an traumatic event.

May **SUPPORTING PTSD RECOVERY** help you or your friend or family member achieve victory with overcoming recovery.

Your friends are here to support you.

Table of Contents

PTSD RECOVERY

Make Our Vets Great Again
and Enable Athletes to
Perform and Recover Faster

Military warriors and civil warriors have much in common. The warriors in the military seek to be the best and often suffer mental and physical damage. Athletic warriors seek to be the best they can be and often suffer mental and physical damage. Concussions, broken bones, and torn ligaments often result in long term bodily and emotional damage.

Similarities in treating trauma for military warriors and civil warrior athletes are virtually parallel. An article by Nolan Peterson about PTSD in the military stated that intense combat experiences he describes as similar to the mental imprinting process that athletes experience when suffering a serious sports related injury like an ACL, broken leg, or concussion. [*What Do PTSD, War Veterans, And Injured Athletes Have In Common*? by Robert Andrews published in *The Institute of SPORTS Performance* May 13, 2016.]

The Investigative Journalist Alan Schwarz fought a battle against psychotropic drugs through his book, ADHD Nation. Schwarz was the author of the book and documentary, Head Game, which brought to light concussions in sports that result in brain injuries, drug abuse and suicidal thoughts. Concussion, the major 2015 motion picture, exposed the NFL coverup that resulted in deaths of some players. Scores of deceased NFL players were found to have brain disease.

In the book ADHD Nation, Alan Schwarz calls ADHD misdiagnosis **"a national disaster of dangerous proportions."** Some legal drugs given to our children are as dangerous as cocaine and have lifelong consequences. He believes that perhaps two-thirds of the childrendiagnosed with ADHD are not ADHD. His book is a damning indictment of the pharmaceutical industry and clearly outlines what is damaging our youth in the name of mental health. Schwarz sees big pharma using academic pressures on our young people and their families.

Of course, big pharma is defending the indefensible and denies the undeniable that children are trading these legal drugs in schools, that there are vast numbers of misdiagnosed cases, and that the CDC could not be right in their evaluations. The CDC reported in 2013 that approximately 6% of U.S. adolescents aged 12 – 19 use psychotropic drugs and 3.2% use antidepressants.

The simple fact is that harmful sugars in food and drinks produce or compound ADHD like symptoms. Another simple fact is that Smart Sugars have a very positive affect while improving brain function. We were excited to participate in a sugar research in Israel with the conclusion that the One Smart Sugar - Trehalose was actually an anti-depressant.

Source and References:

https://www.scientificamerican.com/article/big-pharma-s-manufactured-epidemic-the-misdiagnosis-of-adhd/

Change Your Sugar, Change Your Life http://DiabeticHope.com

http://OneSmartSsugar.com

Expand Your Mind - Improve Your Brain
http://endowmentmed.org/content/view/826/106/

Glycoscience Lesson #48
http://GlycoscienceNEWS.com/pdf/Lesson48.pdf

http://EzineArticles.com/?expert=JC_Spencer

© **The Endowment for Medical Research** http://endowmentmed.org

Note: **GlycoScience Institute** has acquired intellectual properties and assigned to **Texas Endowment for Medical Research, Inc.**

Texas PTSD Veterans Roundtable - Suicide Report

A Glycoscience Lesson from Texas Endowment for Medical Research

by JC Spencer

Texas State Rep. Rick Miller from Sugar Land led Greater Houston Veterans Roundtable on June 8, 2018. Invited to participate, I represented Texas Endowment for Medical Research. The focus was on PTSD and our group discussion was about Mental Health Resiliency.

A director of a PTSD foundation was seated to my left at the Roundtable when he abruptly excused himself from the meeting. We soon learned that a Veteran had committed suicide at their Houston facility.

Wounded warriors shared their stories at the Roundtable that left men and women in tears. These Veterans' stories made an impact on me that verified how difficult it is to get out of the well of depression.

Many people want to help and have heard the Veteran's cry from the well. PTSD is caused by traumatic events that ricochet on and on. Looking down at the Veteran, some throw a bucket into the well. Another throws a rope. Attempt after attempt fails. Finally a Veteran hears the cry and jumps into the well. The vet in the well responds, *"Why did you do that. Now we are both in the deep well."* The rescuing Veteran says, *"I have been in this well before and I know how to get out. We are both getting out"*

Building upon previously published peer-reviewed Pilot Surveys on neurological challenges, the Texas Endowment for Medical Research has established a evidence-based PTSD Pilot Survey program. PTSD is physical and psychological. We address the physical aspect. I told the Roundtable that our desire is to come alongside established organizations that are already helping veterans overcome PTSD.

I have written the book entitled, **SUPPORTING PTSD RECOVERY** and committed to the Roundtable that we will make the ebook version available to every Veteran in America at no charge.

Texas is gaining on California to soon become the #1 state for Veterans with PTSD. Texas counties have different regulations that prevent Veterans from easily obtaining assistance in an adjoining county. Proposed legislation in Austin may change that.

In **Supporting PTSD Recovery** I outline what I believe are the seven most effective methods without psychotropic drugs. To integrate proven methods to conquer PTSD with traditional practice may be acceptable; but to integrate multiple proven methods with Glycoscience proves to be more effective.

We have used the word, "*alternative*" for years. But to the ears of medical professions, the word is combative. Then I used the word, "*complimentary*" for a few years because it was not as combative. However, the word "*complimentary*" rings with the impression that, "*I am better than you.*" After a few more years, I settled on the word, "*integrative.*" When I mentioned this at the Roundtable, the immediate favorable response was, "We will start using that word, '*integrate.*'"

We want to help the doctor be a better doctor by integrating Glycoscience into traditional practice. Let us integrate evidence-based methods to impact the medical and healthcare industry. As one Senator Ted Cruz said, "*We need to tear down the barriers blocking a new era of medical innovation, and the primary inhibitor is the government itself. It's past time to unleash a supply-side medical revolution, so that instead of simply caring for people with debilitating diseases, we cure them ... and embrace a culture of innovation.*"

Throwing buckets of harmful drugs and enough rope to hang yourself into the deep well is not the solution. We are asking Veterans to let Texas Endowment for Medical Research come alongside them so together we can have greater results to benefit more Veterans.

References:

Supporting PTSD Recovery

To Kill A Rat - http://ToKillARatBOOK.com

website: http://TexasEndowment.org

© Copyrighted 2018 by JC Spencer

A Review of How PTSD is Treated or Mistreated Now

Many Current Efforts are Failing.
What if we knew how to improve each current effort?

Post-traumatic stress disorder (PTSD) is a serious challenge to the neurological system. PTSD is triggered by memories of a stressful event that can bring a level of anxiety that can cause intense fear and feelings of helplessness. PTSD can be triggered simply by observing a traumatic event. In fact, symptoms of PTSD may not manifest until months or sometimes years after the traumatic event. It is estimated that more than five million adults in the United States are affected by PTSD each year.

"Experts" are not sure what causes some people to develop PTSD more seriously than others. Your brain processes thoughts and feelings differently from anyone else. Scientists studying the brain observe that there are unique differences in the structure and chemistry each brain. Certain areas of the brain involved with feeling and fear are more hyperactive in some people. This may contribute to PTSD.

Treatments for PTSD often includes:

Conventional psychotherapy or "talk therapy" is one of the main and first courses for PTSD. Another method in addition to traditional "talk therapy" is the use of Cognitive Behavioral Therapy or CBT. CBT focuses on the development of personal coping strategies that target solving current problems and changing unhelpful patterns in cognitions, behaviors, and emotional regulations. This equips the individual with long lasting tools and skills that can be deployed when needed. One main advantage of this form of therapy is that it is generally time limited to approximately 16 weeks which is encouraging to the one seeking help.

Stress management therapy teaches relaxation techniques in an attempt to break the cycle of negative thoughts.

Prayer and meditation can provide a successful breakthrough or crutches and an enabling stumbling blocks when not genuine. Alcoholics and other addicts thrive on foxhole prayers where there is neither commitment nor surrender.

Without question, these treatments when properly administered can be very beneficial; however that may not resolve the issues of PTSD and drastic therapies are called for.

Drastic measures of drug therapies is like throwing dart at the board in an attempt to hit the bull's eye.

The use if psychotropic medications to correct PTSD often causes more problems than solutions.

Drug treatments for PTSD include:

Antidepressants for selective serotonin reuptake inhibitors (SSRIs), including sertraline (Zoloft), fluoxetine (Prozac), fluvoxamine (Luvox), or paroxetine (Paxil).

Benzodiazepines for sedating, including lorazepam (Ativan) and alprazolam (Xanax).

Dopamine-blocking agents (neuroleptics)

Other means of Therapies for PTSD include:

Several mind-body techniques including Eye Movement Desensitization and Reprocessing (EMDR), in which the patient moves his or her eyes rapidly from side to side while recalling the traumatic event. This seems to help reduce distress for some with PTSD. Doctors do not understand how it works or how long PTSD symptoms are reduced using EMDR.

Biofeedback uses the patient's own body signals in an attempt to improve health. Physical therapists may use biofeedback to improve movement in paralyzed muscles. Psychologists may use it to relieve anxiety and help the patient relax.

As the body reacts to stress, the patient learns to perform certain techniques to eventually control the reactions without using the biofeedback machine. Some studies indicate that biofeedback may be an effective treatment.

Hypnosis has been used to treat war-related post-traumatic conditions by inducing a hypnotic deep state so the patient feels safer. Hypnosis is normally used with or by a psychotherapist.

Emotional Freedom Technique (EFT) is a process that combines tapping on acupuncture points while calling to mind traumatic events. Anecdotal evidence with PTSD patients has been encouraging.

Acupuncture has helped with symptoms of PTSD including insomnia, anxiety, and depression.

Nutrition is a do and don't protocol that includes eliminating certain foods which may exacerbate their symptoms as "allergic" might well be another subject altogether. the patient may be allergic. Caffeine causing rapid or increased heartbeat is not necessarily an allergic reaction but a normal bodily reaction to the chemical itself. Certain foods and drinks that fall into this category are stimulants such as coffee, alcohol, tobacco, and too much sugar especially in soft drinks. An improved diet is always welcomed by the body and brain.

Scientists are aiming at the urgent while neglecting the important. Symptoms are treated in impossible efforts to stop the bleeding. The immediate need is understanding what makes our neurological system work, how the signals communicate, and what we can do to improve brain function.

A part of the secret to the neurological system is proper glycosylation of the cells. This can be accomplished through Glycoscience and the application of Smart Sugars technology which is proven to be effective.

**In 2003, Four-Star Marine General Raymond Davis
and I planned to mobilize veterans to declare war
on a domestic enemy, but...**

Psychotropic Drugs to Treat Attention-Deficit/ Hyperactivity Disorder (ADHD) may be Domestic Enemies as are some Drugs used to Treat PTSD.

In 2003, Four-Star Marine General Raymond Davis and I planned to mobilize veterans to declare war on a domestic enemy, but...

General Raymond Davis was America's most decorated hero. His battles were in World War II, the Korean War, and the Vietnam Conflict. Presidents under whom he served included Harry S Truman, Dwight D Eisenhower, John F Kennedy, Lyndon B Johnson, Richard M Nixon, Gerald Ford, George H W Bush, and Ronald Reagan.

In this chapter I will discuss how he and I met and what was to be his next battle. And I will discuss a new battle against a serious domestic enemy to be fought in his name.

Every American Veteran is invited to join and fight this enemy that has millions of Americans in its grasp. The fight is against Post-traumatic stress disorder (PTSD) and psychotropic drugs that often compound the problem.

It is A Time for Truth. It is A Time for Action. It is A Time for Evidence Based Results.

It is time that each of us, including every able veteran, take charge of their own health and demand results instead of acquiescing for someone else to fix the problem.

Ignorance is overcome with knowledge and the wisdom to know what to do with the knowledge. Greed is overcome with a caring heart for others. Mismanagement is overcome with skills that are trained to produce results. Neglect is overcome by leadership with purpose that exchanges greed for compassion and mismanagement with learned skills.

One of the biggest concerns for Veterans is that neurological damage strains the mental and motor skills.

Veterans are Routinely Treated with Toxic Drugs

Our veterans are routinely treated with toxic drugs when new technology is available but not generally used. Four-Star Marine General Raymond Davis and I had a battle plan that was ended when he died of a heart attack on September 3, 2003 at the age of 88.

My good friend Jim Cabaniss, founder of American Veterans In Domestic Defense (AVIDD), introduced me to General Davis. We were excited about his eagerness to champion the cause. He would help save many children by leading the fight and recruiting a volunteer army of veterans.

Today, in memory of General Raymond Davis, we have a new VA cause. Every American Veteran is invited to join our battle against PTSD and we need commanding leaders to fight a domestic enemy. PTSD is to adults what ADHD is to some young people.

Service Medal with three bronze stars; the National Order of Vietnam, 4th Class; the National Order of Vietnam, 4th Class; the Vietnamese Cross of Gallantry with three Palms; two Korean Presidential Unit Citations; the United Nations Service Medal; and the Republic of Vietnam Campaign Medal.

I'm asking every veteran and friends and families of a veteran join forces to fight the Domestic Enemy of Psychotropic Drugs in Honor of General Raymond Davis.

An American Veteran's national campaign against psychotropic drugs was forming in 2003. I was asked to design the campaign with Four-Star Marine General Raymond Davis. The declared domestic enemy was damaging the minds, emotions, and behavior of our children. Our PR campaign would use various action phrases such as: Join General Raymond Davis in his final battle to save America's Children.

General Davis' commanding officers were Truman, Eisenhower, Kennedy, Johnson, Nixon, Ford, Bush, and Reagan.

The campaign for General Davis to lead American Veterans into battle against this domestic enemy would be victorious. Each person in the military have pledged to defend America against every enemy, foreign and domestic.

Abstract of Trehalose Sugar Anti-Depressant Study Now in US National Library of Medicine

May 10, 2013 [update June 2018]*

New research indicates that the Smart Sugar Trehalose has an anti-depressant effect. This discovery may open a new pathway for overcoming stress.

JC Spencer, CEO of The Endowment for Medical Research in Houston, Texas*, said, "*A newly published paper from Israel shows that Trehalose induced an anti-depressant effect in laboratory animals.*" Mr. Spencer has assisted universities and research laboratories in [seventeen]* countries by supplying the sugar Trehalose for further study.

Professor Haim Einat, Ph.D., with the School of Behavioral Sciences, Tel Aviv-Yaffo Academic College, Tel-Aviv, Israel, one of the authors of the paper, told Mr. Spencer, "We are continuing to work on the behavioral and biochemical effects of trehalose and we believe that it might have much potential in our field of affective disorders, both as a possible treatment option and as an additional avenue for us to better understand that pathophysiology and treatment mechanisms in depression. I wish to thank you again for you generous donation of trehalose."

The collaborative effort included Ben-Gurion University in Beersheba, Israel and the College of Pharmacy, University of Minnesota in Duluth, USA.

The study was designed to explore antidepressant and mood stabilizing activity of trehalose in animal models for depression and mania. It is hypothesized that these behavioral changes could be related to trehalose effects to enhance autophagy. Autophagy is a major protein degradation pathway that is essential for stress-induced and constitutive protein folding. Autophagy is the controlled digestion of damaged organelles within a cell and the maintenance of bodily nutrition by the metabolic breakdown of some bodily tissues. It is necessary for the clearance of toxic protein waste especially from neurons. It is believed that to achieve autophagy enhancement is a significant discovery, especially if further studies confirm that indeed trehalose can play a role in human behavioral levels.

Trehalose has long been known for cell membrane protection against stress, health benefits by helping to properly fold proteins, and is effective against neurodegenerative challenges. This study helps explain the pathway these benefits are accomplished.

The Endowment for Medical Research*, a 501 c 3 non-profit research and educational public charity, offers continuing education in the field of glycoscience. A part of their educational program is to make available to the general public free information through www.DiabeticHope.com

The paper was accepted for publication in the journal Psychopharmacology.

The PubMed abstract link is:
http://www.ncbi.nlm.nih.gov/pubmed/23644913

* Note: **GlycoScience Institute** has acquired intellectual properties and assigned to **Texas Endowment for Medical Research, Inc.**

The "Sugar Pill"

*The "Sugar Pill" is an excerpt from the
author's book **To Kill A Rat**.*

The "Sugar Pill" used as a placebo indicates the worthless of regular sugar. However, there is a beneficial category of biological sugars known as "Smart Sugars" found in nature to save and extend your life. Who would have thought that the sugar has the potential to solve some of our greatest health problems?

Smart Sugars are destined to take US to a better future. These sugars can provide healthier children and a reduction in the amount of stress parents feel on a daily basis through improved personal overall health benefits found in these Smart Sugars. Studies verify that these special sugars can support neurological function for those with PTSD, MS, ALS, Parkinson's, Alzheimer's, Huntington's, Stroke, and other nerve function.

The special sugars are the building blocks for glycoforms. Glycoforms are glycan and glycoprotein signal receptor sites on the surface of your cells. Glycolipids operate inside your cells.

What Are Smart Sugars?

These Smart Sugars are operating this moment in your body as your cellular Operating System (OS). Their responsibility is to process all DNA data communication to function, maintain, repair, and replicate. These sugars actually give LIFE to your blood.

Glycoscience (glyco is Greek for sugar) has been hidden in plain sight and is now revealed to radically change how we live. Glycoscience IS the New Frontier of Medicine. This emerging technology will make a major difference in human health. It will do so because the sugars instigate an aggressive attack on viral infections and resistant bacteria.

Big Pharma and our government have already invested billions of dollars in Glycoscience and the general public is still in the dark.

Knowledge of Glycoscience is young. The term "glycobiology" was coined at Oxford University in 1988.

Early in the 21st century, the science of sugars was reconsidered by the *National Academy of Sciences*, the top scientific governmental body in Washington, DC. This prestigious group is made up of Nobel Prize winners and those nominated by Nobel Prize winners.

A distinguished panel of glycoscientists was commissioned for a collaborative effort to explore the future of Glycoscience. The

National Research Council drew from the National Academies: the National Academy of Sciences, National Academy of Engineering, Institute of Medicine. The project was supported by National Institutes of Health, the National Science Foundation, U.S. Department of Energy, the Food and Drug Administration, and the Howard Hughes Medical Institute. Together, they were commissioned to develop the roadmap for the future of Glycoscience. By the close of 2012, the panel published its 200 page report *Transforming Glycoscience - A Road Map for the Future.* Here, they went on record, stating that:

"Glycans impact the structure/function of every living cell in humans, animals, and plants."

The Academy expanded on the importance of the sugars, saying:

"Glycans play roles in almost every biological process and are involved in every major disease"
and
"Elimination of any single class of glycans from an organism results in death."

Another indication of the importance of Glycoscience is found in the bowels of the National Library of Medicine where almost 700,000 references point to research already conducted on some of the most significant life changing biological sugars. The majority of these papers were published within the last few years.

Immunological Testing
Instead of Toxicity Testing

Toxins damage the cellular Operating System (OS) and render it dysfunctional in its ability to properly process data. Toxins alter gene expression and corrupt the body's function to properly maintain, replicate, and repair cells, tissue, and vital organs.

Immunological testing instead of toxicity testing will safely and naturally cover the whole spectrum. Immunity is lowered by the very presence of toxins and renders unnecessary the need to test for toxins.

During the past two decades, I have worked with or studied the work of more than 700 MDs, PhDs, Scientists, Researchers and Educators in the field of GLYCOSCIENCE and Brain Function. During this period I have observed "impossible ailments disappear that standard medical practices cannot address." These catastrophic ailments disappeared through immunology – the modulation of the human immune system. The modulation of the immune system was observed when "Smart Sugars" were supplemented into the human diet.

 an outline of some of the health benefits we have discovered in collaborative efforts with universities in several countries. We have tested the safety and clinical efficacy of certain biological sugars and evidence for the last two decades. <u>The results conclude that several trillions of dollars can be saved through application of Glycoscience.</u>

For example, American veterans can lead the way by using fewer dollars while producing greater results. Using toxin-free biological Smart Sugars we can help relieve human suffering in those experiencing PTSD.

During the last century, the focus has been on problems instead of solutions. Patients, especially those concerned they are experiencing a mental health challenge often put off seeking help. This is often compounded in patience with the fear that such a diagnosis would inhibit or eliminate their current career status or position as is the case in many Veterans PTSDsufferers. Big Pharma knows that the more critical the problem, the greater the opportunity for profit. The focus remains on sickness instead of wellness.

Texas Endowment for Medical Research is helping individuals RECOVER from the flood of health challenges.

Your help is needed to make a difference in the life of individuals who has been accepted in a twelve month Health Recovery Program. This unique program is intended to bring a higher quality of life. Because you care, many others may benefit for generations to come. This evidence-based Health Recovery Program is Toxin Free and focused on improving cellular health and cell communication through glycosylation.

Make a difference – Change a life - Raise a Standard

You can change a life for one while helping many for generations to come.

Co-Partner with Texas Endowment for Medical Research by Sponsoring someone with PTSD. Individuals with PTSD are invited to participatge in a one year Pilot Survey depending on available funding.

Those who donate $25 or more and receive the FREE ebook **To Kill A Rat**
To Kill A Rat *explains how the FDA has used an antiquated approach that restricts attempts to find a cure for any of the 120,000 known diseases. The book explains how the words "treat" and "cure" cannot be used unless the drug kills half the animals in a study.*

In the Pilot Surveys NO DRUGS are used in our Pilot Surveys and no medical claims are made or intended.

Let's Get Started
to MAKE VETERANS GREAT AGAIN

Let us advance the study of therapeutic approaches to PTSD for Veterans so they may be more productive than before and to help others across America.

The Plan:
Without a cost to Veterans, our Plan is to collaborate with other non-profits and corporations to help thousands overcome PTSD.

How:
Bring an awareness of what CAN BE. Woven into the tapestry of **PTSD Recovery** is the awareness of cause and effect and the education of several steps to make significant improvements to what is currently avilable to all PTSD sufferers.

A spokesperson for **Texas Endowment for Medical Research** will be available to speak to all of the Veterans in large groups, small groups, and one on one and to **provide each with a book on PTSD.**

Awareness is detecting the CAUSE for any health challenge and inhibit the compounding of the problem. One major contributor to CAUSE is Sugar and high fructose corn syrup (HFCS). Texas Endowment for Medical Research is working to provide each Veteran with solutions that does NOT compound the problem but helps address PTSD.

The Plan is to provide each Veteran with a month's supply of the healthful sugar. The amount may be determined by the Veteran and his crave for sweets. Each group of ten Veterans may, if they wish, choose a Team Captain to encourage everyone to make today better than yesterday and tomorrow better than today and THIS WILL HAPPEN.

Texas Endowment for Medical Research has assembled the technology to equip and empower American Veterans to help those with symptoms of PTSD to overcome and join the team to help their brothers and sisters in their fight.

Contact JCSpencer@TexasEndowment.org

Outline of Various Support Legs

A five or six legged stool has more stability than a one legged stool. You can balance on a one legged stool for some time but balance you must.

Adding the second leg obviously provides more stability. Adding additional legs may be beneficial but a stool is a rather simple thing, so let's keep it simple while applying the latest and greatest proven technology. You do not have to understand the technology to apply it. For all the scientists who want to know HOW things work – we will provide technical information at the request of each participant, family member, care giver or their medical team as they choose. But, I digress.

I will outline here seven steps. Each of the seven steps alone may be extremely helpful and beneficial. Together the steps can be life changing. **Consider Leg #1**

Step One - Cut off the enemy's supply line

Only Veterans committed to Step One will be considered into the **Texas Endowment for Medical Research PTSD Integrated Program.**

Wars have been won when Step One was followed. Wars have been lost when Step One was not followed. The war to overcome PTSD will require cutting off the enemy's supply line. You must be willing to cut off the enemy's supply line and destroy the arsenal feeding PTSD – Make this commitment and YOU WILL WIN!!!
If you are not willing to make this commitment and will to become accountable to a brother or sister – YOU WILL NOT WIN!!! The people who fail in this program are those who are not committed to take Step One.

During the last two decades, I have observed significant improvements in mental and motor skills as neurological support was applied. We have experienced cases where there appeared to be no hope. We have had teams of doctors tell families to plan funerals – and they had health benefits and lived quality lives.

Begin Step One – Make your own personal list of habits, foods, drinks, or anything you are putting into your body that could be lowering your immune system.
This page is for listing habits, foods, drinks, or anything you are putting into your body that could lower your immune system. Need help? Ask a Veteran brother.

Examples: smoking ____

use of a harmful substance _______________________________________

too many soft drinks ____

not drinking enough water ____

____

____

____

____

____

____

____

____

____

Step Two - Integrating Glycoscience

Glyco is Greek for sugar. Glycoscience is the study of all sugars; the good and
the bad. To learn about Glycoscience is to learn the dangers of regular table sugar and
even worse high fructose corn syrup. While sugar has its dark side, there are several sugars
found in nature that have phenomenally health benefits. We call these beneficial sugars,
"Smart Sugars."

Glycoscience offers Glycan support, circulatory support, nutrition cell support,
mitochondria support, and hormonal support.

Step Three - Hightech Microvascular Circulation Support

Integrate Micro-circulatory application via FDA approved Class 1 medical device.

Microvascular Circulatory Benefits

The capillaries throughout the human body are so fine that blood cells must pass through
in single file. This vast microvascular circulatory system carries nutrients and oxygen to 60
to 80 trillion cells.

We teach three specific methods to achieve improved microvascular circulatory function
without statin drugs.

Learn several way to get more oxygen to the brain.

About 25% of the oxygen we breath is used by the brain.

To safely decrease the resistance to blood flow is an important factor for a healthy brain
and body. Several factors may be integrated to improve the level of oxygen to the brain
and these are presented as part of our education for improved mental and motor skills.

Texas Endowment for Medical Research offers education to Veterans without charge
and actual application for microvascular circulatory improvement as funds are available.

Step Four - Integrate Oxygenation to Counter Oxidation

Several possibilities are available to increase oxygen to the brain and cells of the body. Hyperemic chambers, improved microvascular circulatory function, improved glycosylation of the blood cells, and proper exercise are positive contributing factors.

Step Five - Group support

Step Six - Family and friend support

Step Seven - Spiritual / Prayer support

Spiritual / prayer support is the bedrock into which all others are to be integrated.

See article about my military atheist friend who continually told me, *"There is no God."*

Texas Endowment for Medical Research welcomes collaboration with any organization who wish to SUPPORT PTSD RECOVERY. Our desire is to come along side every Veteran's group and corporation to learn together team building and to discover the ultimate pathway for supporting PTSD. We are listening to all that works and let us make that even better. This is the track on which we choose to run. Let us help each other to help the most. One team building fund raising program we are using is explained on the next two pages.

Veterans may apply for assistance...
SUPPORTING PTSD RECOVERY

Veterans may apply for free or assisted aid designed to improve quality of life. FREE services, educational materials, and products range from minimum maintenance support to urgent Extreme Health Recovery Protocols.

All assistance is drug-free and integrative with your doctor's traditional practice. Your doctor is welcome to monitor and document self-evident health results.

Step by step progress to victory will be clearly outlined. Each veteran will be provided the opportunity to assist his or her fellow veterans in every potential in which they become equipped and the Texas Endowment for Medical Research will supply free education to those who qualify.

Law Enforcement is helping us assist veterans turn Negative situations into empowering Positive results. Improved health begins with the Awareness of Glycoscience so wise choices can be made to overcome the health challenges, especially Neurological Challenges of Mental and Motor Skills. We help connect the dots to achieve "impossible" improvements in mental and motor skills and wish to collaborate with other Veteran groups.

The intent and purpose of Texas Endowment for Medical Research is designed into our efforts for Veterans to receive more than $10,000 worth of benefits in the form of services, education, and assistance for each $5,000 contribution corporate, individuals, and organization contribute to SUPPORTING PTSD RECOVERY.

Several books by the author are available on Amazon and elsewhere: An order from the bookstore at http://TexasEndowment.org helps **SUPPORT PTSD RECOVERY**.

To Kill A Rat

True stories of hope where there was no hope. The book also reveals the secret of why the FDA requires a rat to die to develop a new drug.

$14.97   http://tokillaratBOOK.com

To Kill A Rat is packed with evidence why Glycoscience is the answer to our medical disaster.

The FDA requires millions of animals die to develop new drugs. The FDA uses an antiquated LD_{50} criteria for drug approval. The LD_{50} standard was established to measure just how harmful is any medicine. Lethal Dose 50 requires that all new drugs must kill 50 percent of the subjects in animal studies. Any medicine that cannot establish a LD_{50} level is ruled out from any consideration for FDA approval. This single procedure eliminates toxin free cures from ever reaching the market.

You want your doctor to "Do no harm!" but the medical battle cry of yesteryear was lost to toxic drugs. It is time that is changed. Change is coming and To Kill A Rat explains exactly how the FDA needs to be restructured. A new bill will soon be submitted to Congress and our President intends to sign it. That Bill and the DSHEA Law with suggested amendment are in the book.

Our medical system, designed to mask symptoms, built the road on which we travel today. The ever new toxic miracle wonder drug enabled the doctor and patient to kick the can down the road of sickness. Because of resistant bacteria and viruses that cannot be killed, we are out of both can and road.

During the last century, the focus has been on problems instead of solutions. The medical industry addresses the immediate symptom instead of finding a cure. The drug establishment knows that the more critical and widespread the problem, the greater the opportunity for profit. The focus remains on sickness instead of wellness.

"We need to tear down the barriers blocking a new era of medical innovation, and the primary inhibitor is the government itself. It's past time to unleash a supply-side medical revolution, so that instead of simply caring for people with debilitating diseases, we cure them ... and embrace a culture of innovation." - Senator Ted Cruz

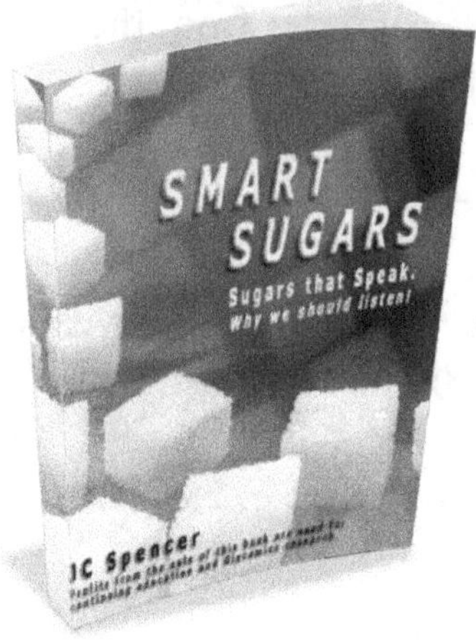

Available on Amazon and elsewhere in various formats including hard bound, paperback, audio, and Kindle. $29.97

For other books on Amazon, search: Smart Sugars JC Spencer

The purpose of **Introducing Smart Sugars** is to provide a starting point for all people to learn about the imminent paradigm shift in medicine and healthcare. Super Sugars are evidence-based and the results are in the irrefutable facts. The emerging data from ongoing research are nothing short of amazing. The future of medicine and healthcare is Glycoscience.

Undeniably, scientists agree that the explosive technological advances in Glycoscience will transform medicine and healthcare. Glycoscience has the potential to dramatically reduce health care costs. Glycoscience is rapidly becoming a part of mainstream medicine and was declared by Massachusetts Institute of Technology (MIT) as "ONE OF THE 10 EMERGING TECHNOLOGIES THAT WILL CHANGE THE WORLD." Working together, The National Institutes of Health (NIH), the Food and Drug Administration (FDA), the National Science Foundation (NSF), the National Research Council, the National Academy of Sciences, the Howard Hughes Medical Institute, and the U.S. Department of Energy (DOE), formed a committee to evaluate the importance, impact, and future of Glycoscience. The group was charged to "articulate a unified vision for the field on Glycoscience and Glycomics" and to "develop a roadmap with concrete research goals to significantly advance the field." We will report on the committee and keep our readers informed with an easy to understand format. It is exciting for these significant agencies to request Glycoscience be taught in high school science classes as well as undergraduate and graduate education. This will assure that future generations will know about the science.

The book provides a glimpse of the Glycoscience of tomorrow and how the future of the human race will be enriched in ways only dreamed of before. The book explains where Glycoscience can take us today and tomorrow. Four FACTS about Smart Sugars Most Smart Sugars are: (1) unknown to the public; (2) are not sweet (some are sweet); (3) extremely beneficial to good health; and (4) the building blocks for the operating system (OS) of the human body. These specific sugars, often called glyconutrients and are unique. Contrary to common thought, glyconutrients are functional beyond just supplying energy to the body. Your body uses these sugar building blocks to construct the actual operating system (OS) of every cell. The sugars and sweeteners consumed by Westerners, such as table sugar (sucrose) and synthetic sweeteners, lower the quality of health and contribute to obesity, diabetes, and other diseases plaguing humans. Bad sugars and sweeteners weaken the immune system and all the other vital functions of the body. The really good sugars, which I call "Smart Sugars" as discussed in this book, can actually help modulate your immune system and balance your hormones which is vital to your health and longevity. Prior to fifty or so years ago our ancestors ate more unprocessed foods and natural sweeteners containing Smart Sugars. Today our foods are depleted of many nutrients and necessary Smart Sugars. It is more important today than ever to supplement our diets with these beneficial functional sugars and with natural vitamins and minerals. The answer to the healthcare crisis is to maintain good health through prevention. A strong, well modulated immune system and well functioning endocrine system are vital to your health and longevity.

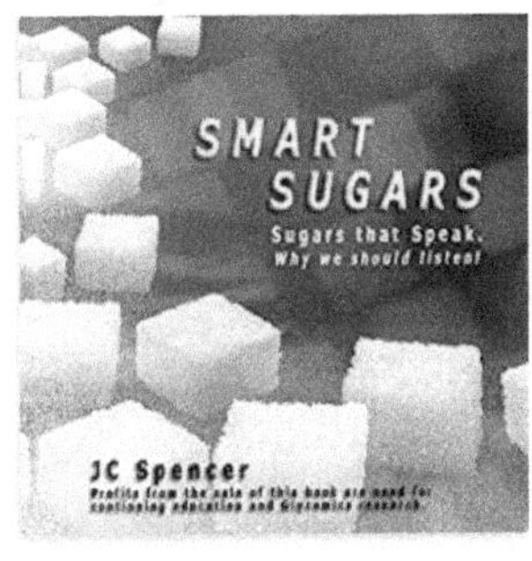

Listen to an audio sample of Smart Sugars on Amazon.

On http://Amazon.com simple request:
JC Spencer Smart Sugars audio

Audible Sample

$49.97

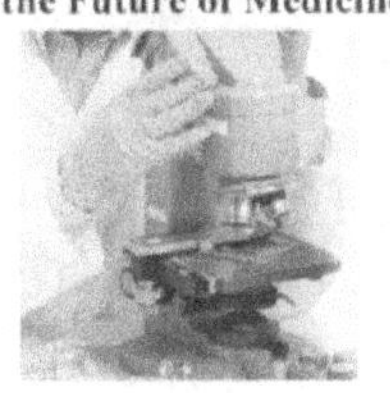

Glycoscience 101 is a collection of over 101 lessons by JC Spencer that explains how Glycoscience will be brought to the people and why Glycoscience is the future of medicine and healthcare.

Glycoscience 101 is not as much of a scholarly study of what is Glycoscience as it is an inside look at the importance of the science and how Glycoscience is more beneficial to human civilization than man has ever known.

Glycoscience, as presented here, is the study of applied biology and chemistry that deals with the structure function of specific carbohydrates which the author describes as Smart Sugars.

Glycoscience 101 conveys an understanding of how Glycoscience impacts all plants, animals, and humans and will change the way we live.

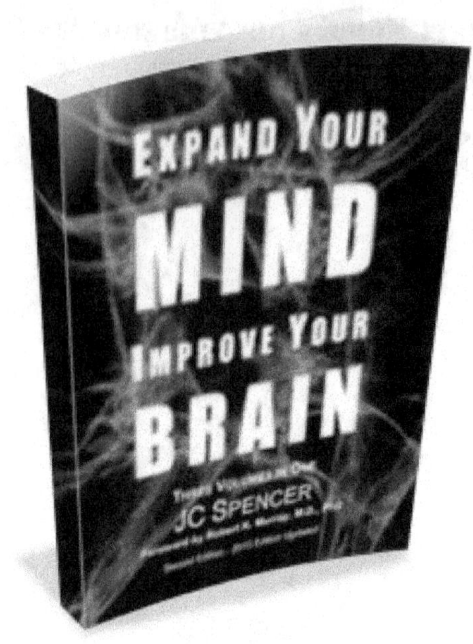

Available on Amazon

This easy to read entertaining science book references over 700 MDs, PhDs, Scientists, Researchers and Educators in the field of Glycoscience and Brain Function.

Available on Amazon and at in the bookstore
Full textbook for a contribution of $197.77
http://TexasEndowment.org

Read why you will want this textbook:
http://www.endowmentmed.org/ExpandYourMind/MindEbook3.html

8.5" x 11" (21.59 x 27.94 cm) 564 pages
Black & White Bleed on White paper
ISBN-13: 978-1482005677
ISBN-10: 1482005670
BISAC: Health & Fitness / Nutrition

The latest in scientific breakthroughs are making it possible to continue further to improve brain function physically and mentally.

Your brain operates on the fuel you supply, be it super food or junk food. The food supply line is for the physical. The mental supply line is super knowledge or junk knowledge determined by the choices you make moment by moment.

This work references well over 700 individuals. I have distilled pertinent knowledge from research by leading professors, doctors, and experts from around the world. Many universities have, within the last few years, established departments or research groups to explore and teach students in the related fields of neural science, glycobiology, glycomics, and mitochondrial research.

GLYCOSCIENCE BOOK SALE

For limited offer, request DISCOUNT code:
Call 281-587-2020 or email jcs@endowmentmed.org

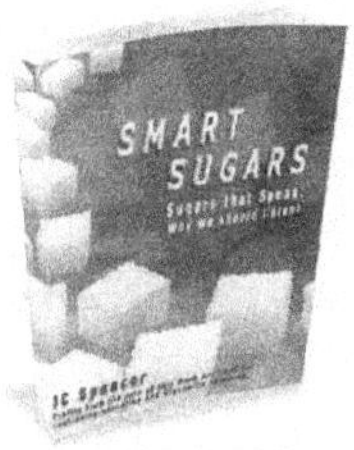

66 pages
Reg Price $29.97

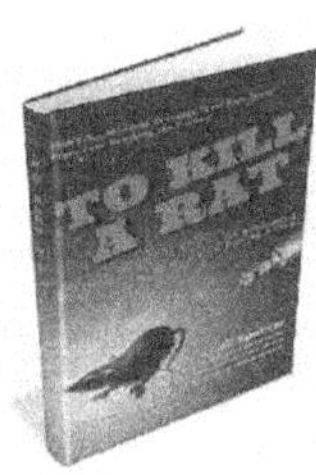

157 pages
Reg Price $19.97

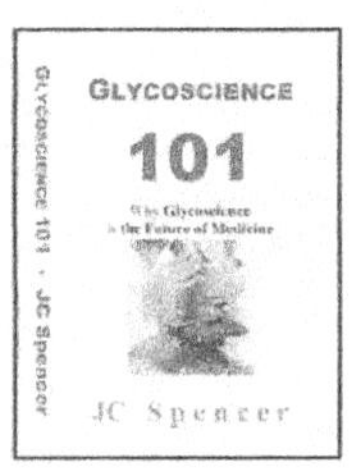

326 pages
Reg Price $39.96

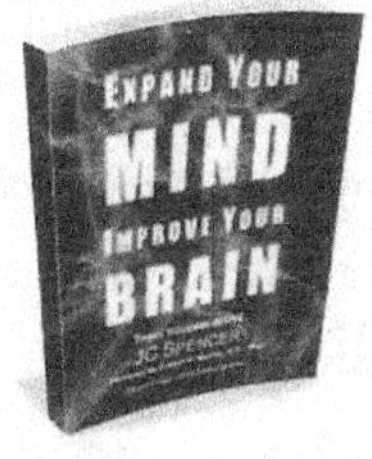

570 pages
Reg Price $129.97

SAVE $75 when you invest in all 4 books for $150 - FREE Shipping

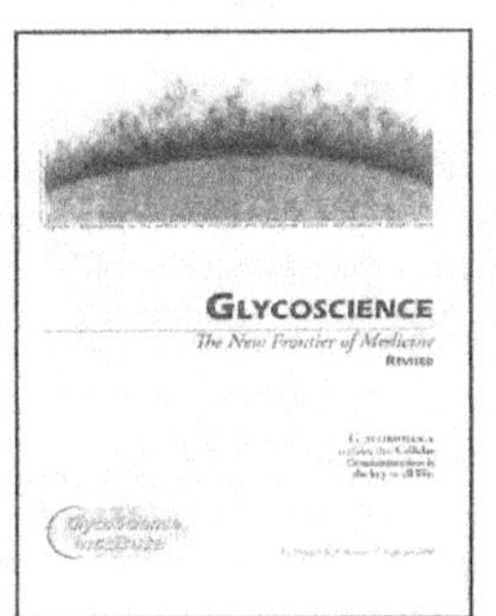

$5

FREE when you purchase all 4 books.

Also available on Amazon world-wide.

For list of other books, type into Amazon search bar **JC SPENCER SMART SUGARS**

Also available in audio and in Kindle.

Help educate others about GLYCOSCIENCE.
http://TexasEndowment.com

Name: _______________________________________

Address: _____________________________________

City: ________________ State: ______ Zip: ________

Phone(s) ______________ Email: ______________

Card #: __________________ Exp: ______ Code ______

Signed: ______________________________________

Amount PAID $____________

Or mail check:

GLYCOSCIENCE INSTITUTE
PO Box 73089 - Houston, Texas 77273 - Office phone 281-587-2020

G Please keep be informed.   Contact: jcs@endowmentmed.org

Closing thought

It is the intent of **Texas Endowment for Medical Research** to come along side other non-profit organizations who are helping Veterans especially those with PTSD symptoms and to provide assistance to achieve optimal results. We will continue to compile documentation toward additional peer-reviewed published reports for helping those with neurological challenges.

Additional References

Additional references and information are provided on our websites and in our other books and publications.

For scheduling speaking engagements or requesting more information contact
JCSpencer@TexasEndowment.org

Texas Endowment for Medical Research's personal Disaster of Hurricane Harvey
Medical records destroyed under six to eight feet of flood water.
NO medical claims are made or intended in any of our evidence based Pilot Surveys.

The worst storm in recent history destroyed years of medical records containing valuable research that can only be replaced by duplicating the research. In 2016 Texas Endowment for Medical Research was given the rights to and possession of vast medical research records that were kept under lock and key in metal file cabinets in compliance with HIPAA Law. Active process was underway to present these finding to an IRB for publication of medical papers when Hurricane Harvey destroyed the research. Over $600,000 is needed to recover the neurological research with advanced Glycoscience technology.

A rich history of Glycoscience discoveries and experience pave the road to the founding of Texas Endowment for Medical Research in 2016. In 2002, The Endowment for Medical Research was founded as, a 501(c)(3) non-profit corporation who collaborated with others to provide four million dollars worth of funding via Smart Sugar products and over 68,000 volunteer hours for the research of improving brain function. From that research, thousands of patients have been helped, and two peer-reviewed papers were published. There was a significant amount of data that had not been processed for publication and was lost during the Houston flood as a result of the devastating effects of Hurricane Harvey. A licensing agreement with GlycoScience Institute was assigned to Texas Endowment for Medical Research for the use and sale of certain intellectual properties including medical research findings and books, published papers, manuscripts, and specific royalty rights to scientific discoveries designed to benefit health challenges especially in the area of neurological conditions.

Our pilot surveys are one way we can work with individuals with unique and /or specific health needs including working with family, caregivers, doctors and nutritionists to monitor changes and progress. These pilot surveys offer both individualized combinations of glyco-enhanced nutrient supplements and with compliant participants can then monitor and extract necessary data for future studies and peer-reviewed reports. The proposed protocols strive to meet and correct a deficiency in glycans. Over two decades there have been a myriad of previous pilot studies that have provided on-going information and our next cohort group of participants are currently applying for inclusion. Much of our funding goes directly into our pilot studies to provide the protocols to a variety of people with differing degrees of health conditions and challenges.

The intent and commitment is to always contribute, to plant, to pay it forward, to help others, and to instill that culture in all we do. When the flood of disaster hit Houston in August 2017 it devastated much but as I told Good Morning America – Houston was not destroyed. We were washed and we will be stronger because of the flood. Digging through the rubble, I know without question VICTORY IS OURS.

This book is dedicated to my dear atheist friend
Everett A. Nichol

August 16, 1927 - December 17, 2012

Everett A. "Nick" Nichol was my friend, a Veteran, and my close confidant for more than 50 years. These are my words spoken at this funeral.

Nick was a close friend and confidant for more than fifty years. His family asked me to conduct his funeral. On December 21, 2012, the winter solstice, end of the Mayan calendar, the day many thought the world would end, I related to family and friends the following:

I loved Nick like a brother for over half a century and yet we were on opposite ends of the political and religious spectrums. Nick and I became friends in 1961 shortly after I returned from a photographic expedition in Africa and moved to Houston from Missouri. He owned a camera store in Pasadena and we worked together for many years processing film, printing giant quality Agfa color photographs for display and publication, and developing scientific breakthroughs in light and color. Nick was what I called a studious perfectionist of color and graphics and a philosophical pragmatist in life.

Nick loved his family of three girls, son, and grandchildren. His son, Don, died in December when he was only 18 and his wife passed one year ago in December. He and Marie were married for 61 years.

In all my years of knowing Nick, I never saw him angry and we never argued. We had many interesting debates but we never argued. Some traumatic event happened when he was a small boy that turned him against God. I mentioned that fact to him which he acknowledged was true, but he never told me nor his family what that event was. It may be that Nick blamed God that his father died when he was only two. But, it was probably a trusted relative that in some way hurt him.

In the late 60s or early 70s, I remember Nick arrived at my home around 9 o'clock and asked me what I had been doing that morning. I responded, "I have been back in our bedroom on my knees praying for you and God has given me assurance and a peace that you will accept Jesus as your personal Saviour before you die." Desiring to immediately change the subject, he pointed to a book on the table and asked what it was about. He pointed to the book "Taste of New Wine" which was written by a Texas businessman and Episcopal layman, Keith Miller. "The book challenges indifference and creates an exciting sense of spiritual renewal and adventure. He doesn't write with religious jargon but he has experienced the real presence of God and has given his heart to the Lord Jesus."

Nick said, "I have been here three minutes and I get all this already." The rest of the day was quite harmonious as we continued on with the business at hand.

One day, he asked me why did I believe the Bible. When I said, "Because I want to.", he replied that he could not argue with that. He thought I was going to defend my position with some long theological dissertation. For more than five decades, he would probe my mind of spiritual matters. He knew that I was not the judge and that I accepted him where he was. We agreed on a lot of things. We agreed that politicians would soon be extinct if they were hemmed in by truth.

After his son died, Nick went to church for a while but soon dropped out. He told me that the reason he did not go to church was that the church was filled with hypocrites. My response to his pragmatic conclusion was, "Nick, if a hypocrite comes between you and God, it only means that he is closer to God than you are."

He explained to me that "religion" is the curse of the planet. I am sure he was shocked at my response, "Religion IS the problem." Then I added, "We should not seek after religion. We are to seek a relationship with the King of Kings and Lord of Lords."

Today we celebrate the life of Nick Nichol. Today is the shortest day of the year, our winter solstice, the day the Mayan calendar ended. It was not because they ran out of stone. The calendar ended on December 21, 2012 because today is a significant day in the heavens. "The heavens declare the glory of God; and the firmament shows His handiwork. Day unto day utters speech, and night unto night reveals knowledge. There is no speech nor language where the voice of the heavens is not heard." (Psalm 19:1-3). Over the years, when Nick would repeatedly declare there is no God, I would point to the heavens and ask him if he thought all that just happened. How many years would you have to shake a box containing all the parts of a watch before a watch would appear?

The universe is a perfectly timed clock from one end of heaven to the other. Nick saw that. I would have loved to have discussed with Nick the significance of this day. The position of the constellations this day was mentioned in the Bible and perfectly matches the Mayan calendar as the end of a cycle and the beginning of the next. We are entering a new time and God is getting ready to do a new work. I do not pretend to understand all that is ahead but we are living in the most exciting time in all history and children will play a significant role in what is ahead.

Woven into our personal relationship was our mutual love for photography, technology, and many things in science in general. Together we developed color technology and implemented it into practice. We developed a lighting technique for color photography that had never been done before. We had lots of fun with it and Nick taught me a new word, "ACTINIC". We developed a lighting technique that was a higher actinic quality than sunlight. With this process we were able to bring out colors in film you could not see with the naked eye. The high actinic quality of light revealed wood grains and oils of master art pieces invisible to the human eye and allowed us to capture that brilliance on film. Nick relished in what we were able to accomplish.

With the light source which we called the "atomic flash" we learned how to capture color and detail in interior and exterior architecture that seemed to break the laws of physics. In truth, we were using an unwritten Law of Light. With one flash, we could light any size building from top to bottom, left to right for hundreds of feet without loss of exposure. For interior pictures, we learned how to light and photograph a room full of objects including tables and chairs without having a shadow behind a single table or chair leg. It was the actinic quality of the light that was more important than the amount of light. The intensity of light, captured on film, immediately in front of the camera was the same as a hundred feet away. To achieve this "impossible feat," only one f-stop would work. And, only one light source flash would work. It was vital that the light go through a tiny precise aperture. And, two sources of light would destroy the image and result in an out-of-focus picture.

Our lighting technique opened many a theological and biblical discussion. "Nick did you know the Bible mentions there are no shadows in heaven? God's Light is the highest actinic quality of perfection. We are but little candles but when the Holy Spirit fills us, the Light in us can reach the whole world."

Nick was strong willed, consistent, dependable, not quick to change, very stubborn, and exercised a level of patience from which we could all learn. He chain smoked and would probably have died a number of years sooner had he not quit smoking. He stopped simply by self-will. He taught me computers and was patient with me when I became frustrated. Before computers, we had a bank of upright electric typewriters operated with pneumatic tubes and the program was a yellow roll of piano paper. To correct an error required Scotch tape and a hole puncher. Together Nick and I pioneered some interesting things in science. Our first mobile phone was rotary dial.

I gave Nick the book, Mere Christianity by C. S. Lewis. He never mentioned if he read it or not. We discussed that C. S. Lewis led J. R. R. Tolkien to faith in Jesus which gave birth to The Lord of the Rings and his other works.

It was perhaps in the 52nd year of our relationship that I told Nick that I felt strongly that his grandmother had prayed for his salvation. He responded, "And my mother."

Sunday afternoon December 16, 2012, I headed to Webster to visit my wife's 97 year old mother. I planned to stop by and visit Nick and perhaps take him out to a nearby restaurant as we had done so many times. We loved to have meals together and had many breakfasts at Kelly's, Denny's, and The Egg & I. One morning as I joined him for breakfast, I said, "Nick, I just learned the secret to all future blessings. Would you like to guess what it is?"

Nick responded, "If I believed, I would say it is, 'Thank you Lord.'"

I started to call Nick on my cell when I noticed that I had missed a call from him. His daughter, Anita, answered the phone and I told her that I was headed over to see Nick. "How is he doing?"

She told me that it was good that I was coming over. He was active even yesterday but had taken a nose-dive after the doctor diagnosed him with advanced leukemia and an eight-centimeter brain tumor. He was not expected to live more than a few hours. His daughter, Nikki, was flying in from Nashville and would be here around 6 o'clock and he was holding on until she got there. I told Anita to tell him I was on my way and for him to wait until I got there.

Nick was setting in a recliner in the living room and was in and out of consciousness. I took his hand. The next hour was precious as Anita, Tony, and I told him he was loved. "It is time for you to ask Jesus to welcome you with open arms," I said. Anita said, "Tony talked with him about that and we believe he has already done that." There was silence to absorb the content of what I just heard.

Then I recalled to him the time I was visiting a Houston medical doctor by the name of John Nance who had suffered a heart attack and was in the hospital. I had told Nick the story before but it was worth repeating at this time.

I asked Dr. Nance if he had ever accepted Jesus as his personal Saviour. He responded, "I'm not worthy." I told him that I wasn't worthy either but salvation is a gift. He said, "But you don't understand. I killed a quarter of a million people. I'm the one who dropped bombs on cities in Germany in World War II and I killed a quarter of a million people. I'm not worthy."

"John," I said, "the thief on the cross certainly was not worthy either but he turned to Jesus as he was dying and said 'Jesus, remember me.'"

As tears streamed down the face of Dr. Nance and my face, he said, "Jesus, remember me." That is how simple it is. God loves us right where we are and he loves us so much that He will not leave us where we are. After recalling this experience to Nick, I hugged his neck and told him how much he was loved. Nikki had just landed at Hobby Airport and would soon arrive. I believe it was at this point that Nick nodded that he knew she was coming to be with him. I wanted to leave so they could be together.

To the daughters I mentioned that Karen and I had given their father the book, "Heaven Is For Real" about Colton Burpo who experienced heaven and returned with many confirming evidences that heaven is for real. Innocent children will lead many into the Kingdom because their words are pure and profound. I asked if Nick had read the book. They said "Yes, he read the book and so did we."

I held Nick's hand in mine and prayed with him and the family, thanking God for the peace and love that filled the room. Providence had brought Nick and me together over half a century ago because of the prayers of a godly mother and grandmother. "Thank you Father for Nick's praying mother and grandmother. Thank you that today their prayers are answered."

Nick rested during the night and breathed his last breath at 8:24 Monday morning December 17, 2012.

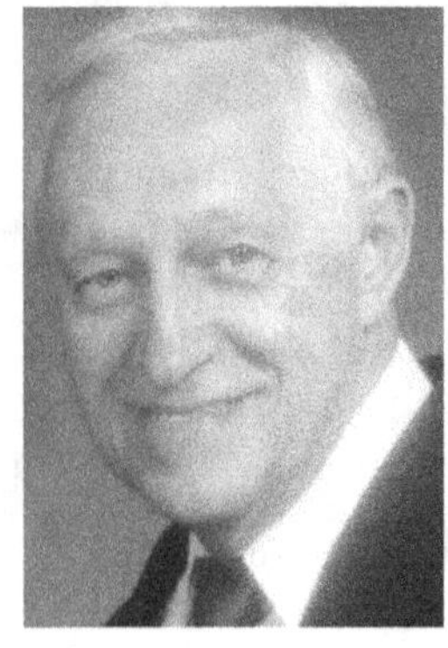

About the Author

JC Spencer is the author of the Glycoscience Whitepaper and has written several Glycoscience books. He has studied the works of more than 700 M.D.s, PhDs, Scientists, Researchers, and Educators in the field of Glycoscience and brain function and collaborated with schools, universities, and research labs in thirteen countries. He has enjoyed international adventures and speaking engagements in many countries. Since the 1990s, he has worked closely with several specialists, doctors, and healthcare professionals in Glycoscience which resulted in the publishing of peer-reviewed papers evidencing improved brain function in Alzheimer's patients, and pilot surveys for various neurodegenerative challenges including Alzheimer's, Parkinson's, Huntington's, ALS, Lyme, Autism, and ADHD. He passionately envisions the field of QUANTUM GLYCOSCIENCE as the proven bull's eye, the Rosetta Stone, the Holy Grail, of medicine and of all healthcare.

JC Spencer is Founder and CEO of the TEXAS ENDOWMENT FOR MEDICAL RESEARCH, Inc, a 501(c)(3) faith-based medical research and education organization and think tank based in Houston, Texas. In collaboration with various organizations, he has conducted surveys on specific biological sugars throughout the United States, Canada, and some foreign countries. He has written extensively about Glycoscience and is also founder and CEO of the GLYCOSCIENCE INSTITUTE.

Mr Spencer and his wife, Karen, have four children, ten grandchildren and five great-grandchildren. They live in Houston, Texas.

You may contact the author
JCSpencer@TexasEndowment.org

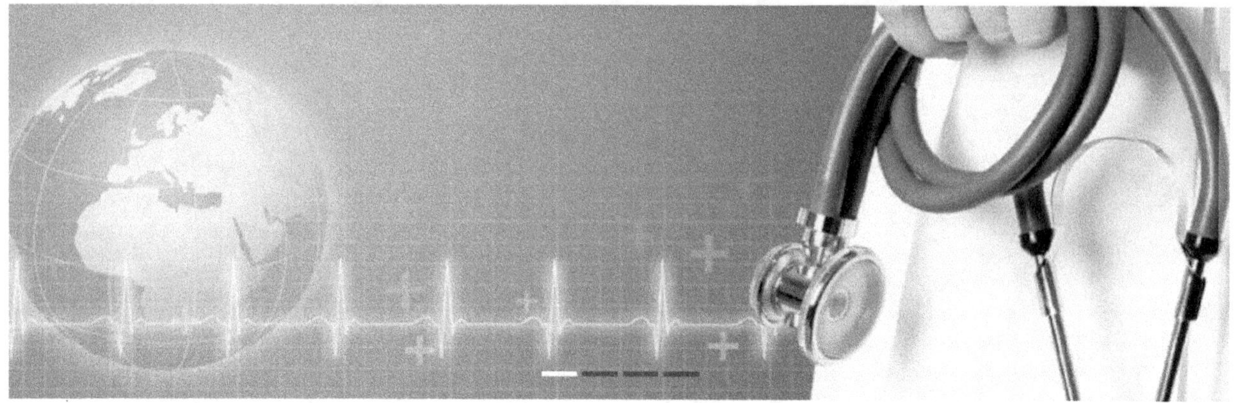

There are bad sugars and there are Smart Sugars. This book is about the Smart Sugars that will change the way we live. "Glyco" is Greek for sugar. "Glycoscience" is the study of sugars, science's relative new term for the discipline of biology that gives life and intelligence to the human race.

PTSD is normally triggered by a sudden traumatic event as may also be the case in other neurological health challenges. A sudden jolt may cause a massive shift in the misfolding of the proteins. It is the misfolding of proteins that impact mental and motor skills.

PTSD is more physical than psychological. Evidence indicates that neurological benefits including the improvement of protein folding may be achieved from specific plant based carbohydrates the author has named Smart Sugars.

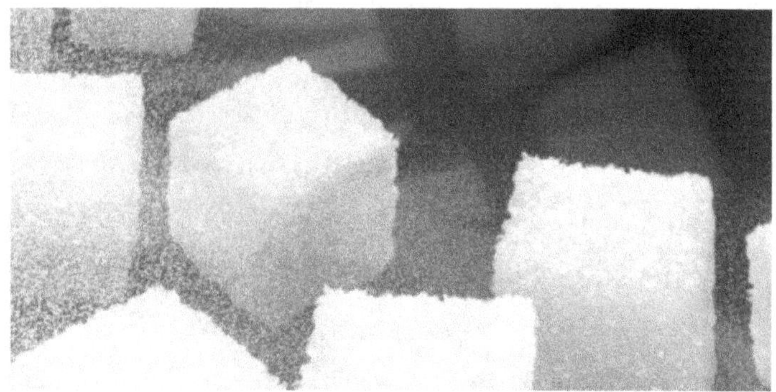

Proceeds from the sale of this book go to further education and research of Glycoscience through GlycoScience Institute, Inc. and the Texas Endowment for Medical Research, Inc., a 501(c)(3) non-profit faith based scientific research, educational, organization.

An educational project of
Texas Endowment for Medical Research, Inc.
PO Lock Box 73089 Houston, Texas 77273
http://TexasEndowment.org

www.ingramcontent.com/pod-product-compliance
Lightning Source LLC
Chambersburg PA
CBHW080247260726
48658CB00008B/3255